The Simple Endometriosis Diet Cookbook:

Nutritious Recipes for Endometriosis Pain, PCOS, Cyst Ovary Syndrome and Fertility.

Copyright © 2024 by Susan Thompson. All rights reserved.

The content, in this book is protected by copyright law. Any reproduction or distribution without written consent from the publisher is strictly prohibited.

The author and publisher have taken precautions to ensure the accuracy of the information provided; however, they do not accept responsibility for any errors or omissions that may occur.

It's important to note that the information shared in this book is for purposes and should not be considered as advice. Readers are encouraged to seek guidance from a healthcare expert before implementing any changes, to their diet or lifestyle.

ISBN: 9798326487926

Table of Contents

Understanding Endometriosis 1
    Symptoms and Impact 1
    Role of Diet in Managing Endometriosis 2
    Goals of an Endometriosis Diet 4

The Basics of an Endometriosis Diet 6
    Anti-inflammatory Foods 6
    Hormone-Balancing Foods 7
    Nutrient-Dense Foods 8
    Avoiding Trigger Foods 9

Key nutrients and functions of nutrients 12
    Benefits of Omega-3 Fatty Acids 12
    Fiber 13
    Antioxidants 14
    Iron 15
    Magnesium 16
    Vitamin D 17

Foods to Include 19

Food to Avoid 26

Breakfast Ideas 36

Lunch and Dinner Recipes 40

Snack Option... 54

Healthy Living Tips for Endometriosis 66

Understanding Endometriosis

Endometriosis is a long-term disorder which manifests as a growth of tissue resembling the endometrium, or the lining of the uterus, in other areas of the body. It may develop from the ovaries, fallopian tubes, the outer layer of uterus and even invade other organs in the abdomen known as the pelvis. These tissues akin to 'endometriosis' undergo cyclical changes during menstruation and are sensitive to hormonal changes leading to inflammation, pain and the formation of scar tissues known as 'adhesions.

Symptoms and Impact

Pain: Some examples include; • Severe pain during menstruation and heavy bleeding • Chronic pain in lower abdomen • Pain during intercourse and deep pain after intercourse • Pain during defecation and during or after urination.

Bleeding: Abnormalities in menstruation such as; Heaviness during menstrual period (menorrhagia) or irregular and long menstrual cycle intercourses.

Infertility: Since endometriosis also impacts the fertility by affecting and scaring the sections in the womb, it causes infertility in some ladies.

Other Symptoms: Topping the list are headache and fatigue; followed by changes in bowel movements such as diarrhea and constipation, bloating, and motion sickness particularly during one's menstrual cycle.

With endometriosis millions of women begin to suffer not only physically, but emotionally and socially as well. The cause of endometriosis is still debated and gives rise to several theories such as retro vaginal flow, genetic endowment, immune influences, and environmental influences.

Role of Diet in Managing Endometriosis

Endometriosis is a chronic condition that affects a significant population of women of childbearing age. Although there is no known medicine that can cure endometriosis completely but diet has an important role to play in controlling the effects of the disease and therefore enhancing the general wellbeing of the patients. An endometriosis diet may help alleviate the symptoms of the disease, regulate inflammation, balance hormones and supply a lot of vitamins and nutrients to your organism.

Inflammation and Diet: Specifically, literature review identified several pathophysiologic factors, including chronic inflammation as a primary cause in endometriosis development. There are items of diet that have effect of increasing inflammation, while there are other foods with anti-inflammatory effects. For instance, consuming a lot of processed foods, sugar, and unhealthy fat, among other food choices, can lead to increased inflammation. On the other hand, some of the foods with low inflammation promoting compounds as the antioxidants, omega-3 fatty acids and other anti-inflamed foods are good for use.

Hormonal Balance: Oestrogen is seen as holding significant responsibility for the development and sustenance of endometrial tissue. An endometriosis diet is a diet that is taken with a lot of care so as to ensure that the hormonal balance in the body is restored by intake of some ingredients such as phytoestrogens, fiber among others.

Nutrient Support: Nourishment is usually a problem for women with endometriosis; their food intake is generally poor, which leads to worse manifestations. Nutrients such as vitamins and minerals are vital for the body's overall functioning and require regular intake; thus, eating a diet with a wide variety of nutrient-dense foods can help ensure adequate intake.

Goals of an Endometriosis Diet

The eating plan aims at improving the condition of endometriosis by managing pains, infertility and other related symptoms that are associated with the disease. The primary goals of an endometriosis diet are to:

Reduce Inflammation: Incorporate foods with medicine tempering properties to help reduce pain that is associated with inflammation and other inflammatory maladies.

Balance Hormones: Avoid certain foods, especially when they contain substances that interfere with handling or processing of estrogen.

Support Immune Function: It should include foods that have nutritional compounds that strengthen the immune system so that the body can have lesser effects of endometriosis.

Enhance Nutrient Intake: Always take balanced diet so as to avoid nutrient deficiencies while at the same time allowing the body to gain the necessary nutrients for a healthy body.

Manage Symptoms: When it comes to the manifestation, understand how specific dietary choices can help with coping with symptoms like digestive ones.

Promote Overall Health: An emphasis has been placed on the interdependent relationships of the three spheres of life's quality: the physique, the psyche, and the spirit.

The Basics of an Endometriosis Diet

There are certain dietary patterns and food that might alleviate the symptoms of Endometriosis and they include; Anti-inflammatory foods that help in eliminating inflammation in the body, eating plenty of nutrients from fresh fruits and vegetables organized together, cutting on processed food that can result in hormonal imbalance, Consuming healthy carbs to increase the nutrient's density in the body, Steer clear of food that is rich in fat as they may cause inflammation to the body. Here are the key components:

Anti-inflammatory Foods

Just as in other cases, the endometriosis sufferers can experience chronic inflammation, which also leads to pain. It is beneficial to include anti-inflammatory foods in your diet plan since it will lead to a lessening of inflammation thus less pain.

Key Anti-inflammatory Foods:

Fruits and Vegetables: These foods are good sources of antioxidants vitamins and minerals, which are all protective against oxidative stress and inflammation. Berries, any green vegetable especially spinach and kale, broccoli, any citrus fruits are ideal.

Omega-3 Fatty Acids: It is commonly present in fatty fish such as salmon, mackerel sardines, flaxseeds, chia seeds, and walnuts among others and has proven a strong anti-inflammatory activity.

Nuts and Seeds: Consuming foods like almonds, walnuts, chia seeds, and flaxseeds help in the selection of healthy fats and antioxidants that reduce the level of inflammation.

Whole Grains: While other grains like white and wheat are detrimental to health and possess inflammation promoting properties, it is recommended to opt for complex grains like quinoa, brown rice, and oats which possess excellent amounts of fiber.

Herbs and Spices: Other spices, like turmeric, ginger, garlic, and cinnamon also provide some potential health benefits like anti-inflammatory effects and antioxidants.

Hormone-Balancing Foods

Endometriosis can be uncontrolled by the use of hormones since estrogen increases it. Propensity to certain types of food has to be taken since it influences hormonal balance.

Key Hormone-Balancing Foods:

Cruciferous Vegetables: Many people regularly consume green leafy vegetables such as broccoli, cauliflower, Brussels sprouts, and cabbage since they contain compounds that assist in the neutralization or metabolism of estrogen in the body.

Fiber-Rich Foods: Any food that is rich in fiber should always be taken since it aids in digestion and can also help the body expel the hormone estrogen through feces since it moves most of the waste products.

Phytoestrogens: Phytoestrogens which are found in foods such as flaxseeds, soybeans and tofu are particularly powerful because they can displace other estrogens in the body and can possibly diminish estrogenic effects.

Healthy Fats: Mediterranean diet consists of healthy fats such as avocados, olive oil, and nuts that are helpful in hormonal balance and the well-being of the body.

Probiotics: Organ meats, wild-caught fish, eggs, whole grains, beans, fermented foods like yogurt, kefir, sauerkraut, and kimchi are essential to the hormone-producing gut.

Nutrient-Dense Foods

It thus becomes useful to adopt a diet that is made up of foods that pack the essential nutrients to ensure that the endometriosis symptoms are well checked and the body's health is boosted. Healthy foods contain vitamins, minerals, and other essential nutrients with little or no sugar, saturated fat, or trans fat.

Key Nutrient-Dense Foods

Leafy Greens: The green-leaf vegetables and fruits such as spinach, kale, and Swiss chard can supply vitamins A, C, E, and K minerals like magnesium, iron and many more.

Berries: The small, dark berries such as blueberries, strawberries and raspberries are becoming prevalent in the market and are important sources of antioxidants, vitamins and fiber.

Lean Proteins: The essential amino acids that can be found in chicken, turkey, and fish are used in improving the state of the body tissues and enhancing the immune system.

Legumes: They are more sources of protein, fiber, iron and many other nutrients such as beans, lentils and chickpeas.

Nuts and Seeds: These are nutrient dense foods that will provide your body with oils, proteins, fiber, vitamins and minerals.

Avoiding Trigger Foods

Some specific types of food are known to worsen the symptoms of the endometriosis disease due to inflammation, hormonal disruption or digestive upset. Thus avoiding these trigger foods can help in managing and combating the effects that are consequent to allergic reactions.

Foods to Avoid:

Processed Foods: These often have unfavourable fats, sugars or additives that may cause inflammation. They consist of such products as processed snacks, fast foods and processed meats.

Refined Sugars: Inflammation and hormonal imbalance: I found that sugar affects the body and can bring inflammation and lead to hormonal imbalance. Inspite of this, one should not take drinks that contain added sugars, candies, baked foods, and other products that have added sugars in it.

Red Meat: Red meat has high saturated fat which means that, it triggers inflammation in the body. It is advisable to take foods rich in these nutrients sparingly, especially by avoiding red meat like beef, pork, and lamb as much as possible.

Dairy Products: Few women also have a penchant for milky foods given the inflammatory contents or the hormonal attributes of such products. It may therefore be important to reduce or even avoid taking milk or cheese as some of the examples of foods that are rich in casein.

Caffeine and Alcohol: Also, both are detrimental to the regulation of hormonal balance and increase inflammation in the body. Avoiding caffeinated items and soft drinks, alcohol, chocolate, and other foods that you find to be irritants may lessen the discomfort somewhat.

Key nutrients and functions of nutrients

It is crucial to stick to a healthy diet when dealing with endometriosis, which is a diet containing the recommended nutrients that our body required. The chemicals that contain antioxidants, relieve inflammation, or help to regulate hormones are vital to wellness.

Benefits of Omega-3 Fatty Acids

Role in Endometriosis: Flaxseed oils contain omega-3 fatty acids which are great anti-inflammatory compounds that may help minimize the inflammation which accompanies endometriosis. They also ensure that hormonal levels are maintained by control of prostaglandin synthesis, for the treatment of dysmenorrhea.

Sources:

Fatty Fish: Examples of fish that are fatty acids boosts includes salmon, mackerel, sardines as well as trout.

Flaxseeds and Chia Seeds: These seeds can blend easily with butters, yogurts, smoothies, oatmeal, and salads.

Walnuts: A tasty snack that can also give consumer the benefits of these special omega-3 fatty acids.

Algal Oil: An alternative source of supplement this is for vegetarians and vegans particularly a plant-based supplement.

Benefits:

Reduced inflammation and pain.

Improved hormonal balance.

Enhanced overall cardiovascular health.

Fiber

Role in Endometriosis: Fiber is useful in flushing out of the over produced estrogen hence playing a pivotal role in hormonal manageability. It also supports the digestive system, that should be helpful for individuals experiencing digestion problems that are linked to endometriosis.

Sources:

Fruits: Synopsis An essay about different types of fruit produced includes: apples, pears, berries, and oranges.

Vegetables: The cruciferous vegetables include broccoli, Brussels sprouts and cauliflowers; the orange veggies include carrots while the green leafy vegetables include kale and spinach.

Whole Grains: Oats, quinoa, rice, and barley are all examples of grains that can be included in a healthy diet.

Legumes: And we are talking about lentils, chickpeas, black beans, and kidney beans that can be consumed in large quantities or as a vegan protein.

Benefits:

Promotes regular bowel movements.

Aids in the elimination of any surplus or toxic estrogen within the body.

Supports overall gut health.

Antioxidants

Role in Endometriosis: Aim: Antioxidants reduce oxidative stress which is typically increased in endometriosis and can propagate inflammation and tissue injury. Yet, antioxidants are reducing agents that are able to counteract free radicals as to prevent cell damage and inflammation.

Sources:

Fruits: Blueberries, strawberries, raspberries, and probably all types of citrus fruits.

Vegetables: Cruciferous vegetables, green leafy vegetables, and red fruits and vegetables.

Nuts and Seeds: The nuts and seeds that people preferred know are almonds, sunflower seeds, and pumpkin seeds.

Herbs and Spices: Here are the medicinal foods – Turmeric, ginger, garlic, cinnamon.

Benefits:

Decreased undesirable generation of free radicals and some plasma inflammatory markers.

Protection of cellular health.

This may be in the form of pain relief and other uncomfortable symptoms that may be related to the condition.

Iron

Role in Endometriosis: This metal live is important in the production of haemoglobin which aids in the transfer of oxygen in the bloodstream. Endometriosis patients displayed anaemia because of heavy blood flow during menstruation, which was observed as heavy menstrual bleeding.

Sources:

Red Meat: Some meats such as beef, lamb and pork with a minor inclusion of pork due to its inflammatory properties were consumed.

Poultry: Chicken and turkey.

Fish: Sardines and salmon.

Plant-Based Sources: Lentils Spinach Fortified Breakfast cereals (with calcium) Tofu (absorption is boosted when consumed along with Vitamin C).

Benefits:

Prevention and treatment of anemia.

Improved energy levels and reduced fatigue.

Enhanced overall health and well-being.

Magnesium

Role in Endometriosis: Ever since, the mineral has been shown to be too essential in the relaxation of muscles, decrease in pain sensations among others. It can deal with the menstrual cramps and it can also help to reduce the stress level and improve the sleeping pattern which is important for the patient suffering from endometriosis.

Sources:

Leafy Greens: Spinach, Swiss chard, and kale are examples worth using when describing the differences between the meal types.

Nuts and Seeds: There are several types of seeds, for example, almonds, pumpkin seeds, and sunflower seeds.

Legumes: These are the sorts of foods: black beans, chickpeas, lentils

Whole Grains: The better options include brown rice, quinoa, and whole wheat bread.

Benefits:

Muscle relaxation for reduction of muscle cramps and relief of pain during menstruation.

Better ways of dealing with stress and stress-related disorders.

Improved sleep quality.

Vitamin D

Role in Endometriosis: Vitamin D is important for body immune modulating feature and has antioxidant effects. It is important to maintain sufficient levels of vitamins within the body because they play a crucial role for a person's well-being, including the possible alleviation of the symptoms associated with endometriosis.

Sources:

Sun Exposure: One of the last types of vitamins that we need for our body is vitamin D, which is synthesized in the skin through the exposure to sunshine.

Fatty Fish: Their opp one is made of seafoods like salmon, mackerel, and tuna.

Egg Yolks: Vitamin D is available in certain fish, therefore consuming fish regularly is good for the body.

Fortified Foods: Juice milk, and fruits for breakfast; orange juice, greetings and good morning; Cereals, greetings and good morning for breakfast.

Benefits:

Enhanced immune system function.

Reduction in inflammation.

This may lead to an improvement in mood and energy which makes it more preferable than alcohol.

Foods to Include

Endometriosis diet is a concept that involves eating foods that fight inflammation, balance hormones and contain vital nutrients. Some of these foods can include; There are many ways of a variety of these foods which could assist control of the symptoms and enhance the health.

Fruits & Vegetables

Importance: Fruits and vegetables are known to contain vitamins, minerals, antioxidant group of substances and fiber. As mentioned before these nutrients assist in fighting inflammation, regulating hormonal management and providing nourishment.

Recommended Foods:

Leafy Greens: That is because green leafy veggies such as spinach, kale, Swiss chard, and arugula.

Cruciferous Vegetables: Sr: Broccoli, cauliflower, Brussels sprouts, cabbage.

Colorful Vegetables: Bell peppers, carrots, sweet potatoes, and beets As you are well aware, vegetables come in many varieties and sizes and can be eaten raw or cooked.

Berries: The wild types of berries that could commonly be found are the blueberries, strawberries, and raspberries, and blackberries.

Citrus Fruits: Oranges, grapefruits, lemons, and limes: These fruits are known to be very nutritious for the body.

Benefits:

high in the content of antioxidants and anti inflammatory substances.

A naturally healthy snack source, containing fibre to aid digestive system.

The basic vitamins and minerals have to be supplied to fulfill the nutritional needs of the body's vital organs which are part of our systems.

Whole Grains

Importance: Whole grains provide the beneficial combination of fibres, vitamins, and minerals and should be consumed daily. It helps in regulation of hormones and the energy is more enduring.

Recommended Foods: Quinoa: This bean is a good source of protein and it has more fiber content.

Brown Rice: Both fiber and B vitamins can be obtained from this type, in order to maintain a healthy diet.

Oats: High content of fibre and nutritious for the heart.

Barley: Many contain high fiber content and several other nutrients that are necessary for the body.

Whole Wheat Products: Whole grain bread, pasta, and cereal products Whole grain foods that are low in fat are good sources of fibre and can decrease the risk of cardiovascular disease when eaten in moderation.

Benefits:

Resist the conversion of testosterone into estrogen, thus helping in the removal of excess estrogen.

They should be able to supply long lasting energy to the body to avoid surge in blood sugar levels.

Support digestive health.

Lean Proteins

Importance: Protein is required by the body to provide support for the tissues, to maintain muscle mass and for various other activities. Lean proteins afford these benefits without the fats that cause inflammation to occur in the body walls.

Recommended Foods:

Poultry: Chicken and turkey.

Fish: Canadian focusing on (salmon), Spanish (mackerel, sardines), and rainbow trout.

Legumes: These include lentils, chickpeas, black beans, kidney beans and many others.

Tofu and Tempeh: Sources of proteins which are plant derived and which contain all the nutrients that the body needs.

Benefits:

Stimulates the healing of damaged tissue and has positive effects on muscular system.

There are vitamins and minerals that should be included in any diet plan.

Support overall metabolic health.

Healthy Fats

Importance: Essential fatty acids are needed for effective hormone synthesis, anti-inflammation, and the general health and functionality of the cells. That minimizes occurrences of hormonal fluctuation and offers sustained energy supply.

Recommended Foods:

Avocados: Low in saturated fats and packed full of the powerful plant compounds like fiber.

Nuts and Seeds: Such nuts as almonds, walnuts, and seeds like flaxseeds, chia seeds, and sunflower seeds.

Olive Oil: Nutritionally beneficial due to the presence of monounsaturated fats and antioxidants.

Fatty Fish: Omega-3 fatty acids can be found in fatty fish such as salmon, mackerel and sardine.

Benefits:

Influence the synthesis of the hormones and keep the proper hormonal levels.

Reduce inflammation.

Ensure adequate amounts of fats for the body wellbeing.

Maintaining health and wellbeing.

Contain fats that are important for the general wellbeing of the body.

Herbal Teas and Natural Remedies

Importance: There are some more recommendations for women who suffer from endometriosis and wish to minimize its impact on their lives: Some of the herbs possess characteristics such as inflammation reducers and aids in balancing hormone.

Recommended Teas and Remedies:

Ginger Tea: Helps to decrease inflammation and provide relief to those who have upset stomachs.

Turmeric Tea: It contains curcumin which is a potent anti-inflammatory agent, among many other benefits.

Green Tea: Rich in antioxidant compounds and might also aid in reduction of inflammation.

Peppermint Tea: Aids in digestion and decreases stomach swelling.

Chamomile Tea: It is relaxing and is used in easing stress and tension of the muscles.

Benefits:

Will offer anti-inflammatory and antioxidant advantages.

Promote digestion and decrease gastrointestinal issues such as bloating, constipation, and gas.

Used for the promotion of relaxation and combat of stress.

By consuming food high in these nutrients and ensuring a diet rich in nutrient dense foods, those with endometriosis can alleviate symptoms and promote general well being. An endometriosis-friendly diet not only considers the disease's-related issues but also focuses on a healthy lifestyle for the patient.

Food to Avoid

For patients with endometriosis, they should avoid these foods in order to minimize their effects on this condition and general wellbeing. These foods can trigger inflammation, hormonal imbalance, and exacerbate the digestive symptoms that are often experienced with endometriosis.

Processed Foods

Why to Avoid: Junk foods contain bad fats, sugars, and chemicals that can cause inflammation and disrupt hormones in the body. They contain very little amounts of essential nutrients, but they are rich in calories thus leading to weight loss and other hormonal related issues.

Common Processed Foods:

Processed and convenience foods such as chips, crackers, cookies, etc.

Fast food

Cured meats and sausages (hot dogs, sausages, deli meats)

Frozen entrees and fast foods

Candy-like cereals and snack bars

Negative Impacts:

Inflammation: Most manufactured foods include trans fats and refined oils these are some of the most aggressive inflaming agents.

Hormonal Disruption: This includes the effects of additives and preservatives which interferes with the normal hormonal balance in the body.

Nutrient Deficiency: These foods do not contain nutrients most needed by the body and thus, lead to malnutrition, which may worsen endometriosis symptoms.

Digestive Issues: One of the biggest disadvantages of processed foods is that they contain high amounts of sodium and low amounts of fiber, which result in bloating and constipation among other symptoms.

Refined Sugars

Why to Avoid: Added sugars can also cause inflammation, interfere with stabilizing blood sugar levels, and potentially disrupt hormones. Junk food lacks nutritive value and is characterised by additives which results in excessive weight and hormonal imbalances.

Soft drinks (Coca cola, Effect, commercial juices, energy drinks)

Sweets (cakes, cookies, pastries, candies, chocolates), treats

The primary sources are sweetened breakfast cereals and granola bars

Meal's accompaniments (ketchup, barbecue sauce, salad dressing, etc.)

Snack foods (cracker/ flavoured yogurt etc)

Negative Impacts:

Inflammation: Increased sugars contribute to enhanced inflammation levels in a body.

Hormonal Disruption: Oscillations of blood sugar levels cause changes in the body's ability to respond to insulin, which is a branch of hormonal regulation.

Energy Spikes and Crashes: Sweet foods produce high fluctuations of the blood glucose levels coupled with low energy levels and erratic moods.

Increased Pain: Some of the likely causes for enhanced menstrual pain as well as other signs of endometriosis include inflammation and hormonal fluctuation.

Red Meat

Why to Avoid: Achieving a low glycemic diet is simple since it only need to avoid excessive red meat especially if processed or contain a high fat. It also contains arachidonic acid the raw material for formation of inflammatory prostaglandins in the body.

Common Sources of Red Meat: Common Sources of Red Meat:

Beef (steaks, burgers, roasts)

Pork (chops, bacon, sausages)

Lamb

INSTANT DELI PRODUCTS (salami, ham, hot dog)

Negative Impacts:

Inflammation: Another realized reason associated with the consumption of red meat is that it contains high levels of saturated fats which causes inflammation.

Hormonal Disruption: Red meats are known to sometimes have added hormones or residues of hormones from feed and these can interfere with human hormones.

Digestive Issues: Some negative side effect that is usually associated with the red meat despite its rich content in protein is that it causes a lot of problems in digestion meaning that it can lead to stomach upsets, bloating and even constipations.

Increased Risk of Endometriosis Flare-ups: Unfortunately, red meat contains some compounds which are actually inflammatory and which make endometriosis symptoms worse.

Dairy Products

Why to Avoid: Different people with endometriosis may experience challenges consuming diary products because some of the products cause inflammation as well as upset stomachs. They may also contain hormones that can alter balance of hormones within the body and lead to severe health complications.

Common Dairy Products:

Milk

Cheese

Yogurt

Butter

Ice cream

Negative Impacts:

Inflammation: Protein, which is present in the dairy product also has casein and lactose which might cause inflammation or digestion problems in some people.

Hormonal Disruption: Cheese and yoghurts, for example, contain natural hormones and other hormones are added in the processing of the products.

Digestive Issues: Lactose intolerance is not a fancy ailment, and dairy for most people causes bloating, gas, and diarrhea.

Potential for Increased Symptoms: Sensitive stomach is a sound reason behind choosing not to consume dairy since it increases inflammation and enhances the condition of endometriosis.

Caffeine and Alcohol

Why to Avoid Caffeine and Alcohol and There Effects on the Human Body

Caffeine can cause inflammation, hormonal imbalance, and affect the gastrointestinal tract while alcohol may worsen the symptoms of endometriosis due to its inflammatory properties. These substances should be avoided or their intake should be controlled to some extent in order to prevent and alleviate the symptoms.

Caffeine

Impact on Endometriosis: Caffeine contained in coffee, tea, sodas, and energy drinks also affects the central nervous system, raises the levels of stress hormones, which can be detrimental to the patient's condition.

Common Sources of Caffeine:

Coffee

black tea, green tea, and selected herbal teas

Soft drinks and colas

Energy drinks

Chocolate and cocoa products

Negative Impacts:

Hormonal Imbalance: Caffeine has been shown to raise cortisol levels and thus disrupt the natural hormonal cycle and potentially affect estrogen levels.

Increased Pain Sensitivity: Caffeine can possibly make one more sensitive to pain because it is a stimulant of the central nervous system.

Digestive Issues: Caffeine is a diuretic that can cause dehydration and has been noted to cause or worsen constipation, which is highly prevalent in people with endometriosis.

Sleep Disruption: Caffeine is known to disrupt the natural sleep-wake cycle and therefore can lead to poor quality sleep, and sleep is very important for chronic pain and inflammation.

Recommendations:

Limit Intake: It is important not to quit caffeine consumption all at once because it can lead to withdrawal symptoms. Limit your intake of coffee or other types of caffeinated products to not more than a cup in a single day.

Switch to Alternatives: Replace liquid caffeine with caffeine-free herbal teas, including chamomile or peppermint for relaxation or digestion respectively.

Alcohol

Impact on Endometriosis: Ethanol influences estrogen, which in turn can cause imbalance in liver enzymes that are necessary for hormonal excretion and inflammation. This is especially true when one is used to the regular consumption of alcohol as this can lead to poor health and weakened immunity.

Common Sources of Alcohol:

Beer

Wine

Aperitif wine, Brandy, Gin & Tonic, Vodka & Juice, Business Lunch Beer, Business Lunch Wine, Whiskey & Coke

Cocktails and mixed drinks

Liqueurs

Negative Impacts:

Hormonal Imbalance: They entail that ethanol consumption leads to a hormonal change that precipitates estrogen, this in turn leads to the growth of the uterine lining, endometrial tissue, outside the uterus.

Liver Stress: The specific tissues affected by the hormones are the liver, which synthesizes and eliminates unused hormones from the bloodstream. Sex hormones include estrogen, and alcohol affects this hormone by damaging the liver, and therefore the hormones accumulate.

Inflammation: Some cognition is that alcohol calls for fats close to the human body's inflammation indicators and might make the twinges of pain and other publication symptoms of endometriosis worse.

Immune System Suppression: Alcohol intake has been regarded as having adverse effects on the immune system, thus making the body of an individual with endometriosis or other diseases more vulnerable when regularly consumed.

Recommendations: Limit Intake: In case you enjoy alcohol, moderate or avoid regularly, and consume it occasionally only in special occasions, do not exceed one drink per day.

Choose Wisely: Instead of alcoholic drinks, prefer wines or light beers; however, opt for high alcohol content mixed drinks and liquor.

Hydrate: Alcohol should be taken in moderation, but most importantly, one should drink water in between and after taking alcohol to help his/her body detoxify it.

Breakfast Ideas

1. Chia Seed Pudding

- Ingredients: 3 tablespoons chia seeds, 1 cup almond milk, 1 teaspoon vanilla extract, 1 tablespoon maple syrup, fresh berries to garnish.

- Instructions: Mix chia seeds, almond milk, vanilla extract, and maple syrup in a bowl. Mix gently, then chill for at least 12 hours. In the morning, garnish with fresh berries.

2. Green Smoothie

- Ingredients: Spinach – 1 cup, Banana – 1/2, Avocado – 1/2, Unsweetened almond milk – 1 cup, Flaxseeds – 1 tablespoon, Ice cubes.

- Instructions: Mix all ingredients until creamy. Serve immediately.

3. Oatmeal with Berries and Nut

- Ingredients: Rolled oats ¼ cup, water or almond milk 1 cup, mixed berries ½ cup, chopped almonds 1 tablespoon, honey 1 teaspoon.

- Instructions: To prepare the oats, cook as per the instructions written on the packet or box. Serve with a topping of berries, almonds and honey.

4. Avocado Toast

- Ingredients: Whole grain bread, avocado, sea salt, red pepper flake, pumpkin seeds.

- Instructions: Prepare the bread by toasting it. Crumble the avocado and spread it on the toast. Season with salt, red pepper and pumpkin seeds.

Overnight Oats

Ingredients:

1/2 cup rolled oats

1 cup unsweetened almond milk

1 tablespoon chia seeds

1/2 teaspoon cinnamon

1/2 cup mixed berries

1 tablespoon almond butter

Instructions:

In a jar or a container, mix the oats, almond milk, chia seeds, and cinnamon.

Mix thoroughly, cover and let it stand in the refrigerator for about 12 hours.

For breakfast, spread mixed berries and almond butter over the top before consuming.

Sweet potato breakfast bowl

Ingredients:

1 medium sweet potato (baked or roasted)

1/2 cup Greek yogurt (optional for dairy-free)

1 tablespoon almond butter

¼ cup low-sugar granola

1 tablespoon hemp seeds

Instructions:

Peel and mash the baked sweet potato and put it in a separate bowl.

Top with greek yogurt, almond butter, granola and hemp seeds.

Enjoy it warm or at room temperature.

Lunch and Dinner Recipes

Quinoa salad with Vegetables The recipe for the quinoa salad with vegetables will be detailed below.

- Ingredients: 50 g quinoa, cooked as per instructions on the packet 120 g cherry tomatoes, halved 150 g cucumber, diced 60 g red onion, finely diced 60 g feta cheese, crumbled 2 tbsp olive oil 1 tbsp lemon juice Salt and freshly ground black pepper.

- Instructions: In a big bowl, mix the cooked quinoa with tomatoes, diced cucumber, finely chopped red onion, and crumbled feta cheese. Finally, carefully pour liquid olive oil and lemon juice over it. Mix with salt and pepper season. Toss to combine.

Salmon baked in the oven accompanied by asparagus.

- Ingredients: 2 medium sized salmon fillets, 2 bunches of asparagus (with ends trimmed), 2 tablespoons olive oil, half a lemon (cut into wedges), 2 cloves of garlic minced, black pepper and salt.

- Instructions: Melt butter and combine it together with honey. In another bowl arrange all blend ingredients: Cream of Tartar, Baking Soda, baking powder and cocoa powder.

Preheat your oven to 375°F (190°C). Organizing main ingredients: Arrange salmon and asparagus on a baking sheet for roasting. Season with sea salt and paved with olive oil then garnish it with lemon slices and minced garlic. Sprinkle with salt and pepper, to each person's preference. Bake for 20 minutes or until salmon is cooked through.

Lentil Soup

- Ingredients: 1 cup dried lentils, 1 chopped onion, 2 chopped carrots, 2 green stalks of celery chopped, 2 minced cloves of garlic, one can diced tomatoes, 4 cups vegetable broth, 1 tsp cumin, 1 tsp paprika, salt, pepper to taste.

- Instructions: In a large pot over medium heat add olive oil, onion, carrots, and celery, which need to be cooked until softened. When the oil is sufficiently hot, add the minced garlic and cook for another one minutes. Bring lentils to a simmer, tomatoes, vegetable broth, cumin, and paprika. Now, to a boil, and then to a low heat and let it bubble for about 30 minutes or to the tenderness of the lentils. Use salt and pepper on the season.

Chickpea and Spinach Stir-fry

- Ingredients: You will need: 1 can chickpeas (drained and rinsed), 4 cups spinach, 1 onion (chopped), 2 garlic cloves (minced), 1 tablespoon olive oil, 1 teaspoon cumin, 1 teaspoon turmeric, salt and pepper to taste.

- Instructions: In a pan, heat olive oil over medium heat. For the sauce, sauté onion and garlic until they turn to brown. Stir in the chickpeas, cumin and turmeric. Cook for 5 minutes. Add spinach and stir until it wilts. Season the food with salt and pepper.

Stuffed Bell Peppers

Ingredients:

4 bell peppers of any color

1 cup quinoa (cooked)

1 can black beans (drained and rinsed)

1 cup corn kernels fresh or frozen

1 cup diced tomatoes

1 teaspoon cumin

1 teaspoon paprika

Salt and pepper according to taste

1/4 cup chopped fresh cilantro

1 avocado (sliced, for garnishing)

Instructions:

Before continuing, it is helpful to preheat the oven to 375 degrees Fahrenheit (190 degrees Celsius).

Trim off the tops of the bell peppers and scoop out the seeds and the membranes.

In a bowl, mix in the cooked quinoa, black beans, corn, tomatoes, cumin, paprika, salt and pepper.

Continue to fill the bell peppers with the quinoa mixture.

Arrange the stuffed peppers in a casserole, cover with foil and bake for 25-30 minutes.

The foil should be removed and the dish should be baked for an additional 10 minutes.

Garnish with fresh cilantro and avocado before you are ready to serve the dish.

Endometriosis Benefits: It is packed with fiber, plant protein and antioxidants. Quinoa and black beans are sources of amino acid, and bell peppers and tomatoes are also packed with vitamin and antioxidants.

Zucchini noodles with pesto and cherry tomatoes

Ingredients:

4 medium zucchinis (sliced into thin ribbons to mimic noodles).

1 cup cherry tomatoes – halved

1/2 cup basil pesto (preferably homemade, but store bought is okay too)

1 tablespoon olive oil

Salt and pepper to your desired taste.

2 tablespoons pine nuts (optional for garnish)

Instructions:

In a large skillet, heat olive oil at medium heat.

Fold in the spiralized zucchini noodles and continue to cook for 2-3 minutes until it is slightly tender.

Throw in cherry tomatoes and stir for an additional 2 minutes.

Turn off the heat and mix with pesto.

Season with salt and pepper to your preference.

If preferred add the pine nuts on top of the dish.

Endometriosis Benefits: Zucchini noodles are low in carbohydrates but high in fiber compared to the regular pasta while the basil pesto provides essential fats and fight inflammation. Cherry tomatoes add antioxidants.

Coconut curry with chickpeas and spinach

Ingredients:

1 tablespoon coconut oil

1 onion (chopped)

2 garlic cloves (minced)

1 tablespoon ginger (minced)

1 can chickpeas (drained and rinsed)

1 can diced tomatoes

1 can coconut milk

2 cups fresh spinach

1 tablespoon curry powder

1 teaspoon turmeric

A pinch of salt and pepper for seasoning

Cooked brown rice, to serve

Instructions:

Melt coconut oil in a large pot under medium heat.

Throw in the onion, garlic and ginger and fry until brown and soft.

Stir in curry powder and turmeric and then let it cook for another minute.

Mix in chickpeas, diced tomatoes, and coconut milk. Bring to a simmer.

Bake in the preheated oven for 15- 20 minutes with the ingredients intermingling.

Stir spinach in and simmer until it is wilted.

Season with salt and pepper, to your liking.

Serving suggestion: Serve over cooked brown rice.

Endometriosis Benefits: Coconut milk has a good amount of healthy fats and next to it, chickpeas are also filled with protein. Spinach contains iron and magnesium that are essential in providing energy and muscle movements.

Baked cod with lemon and fresh herbs.

Ingredients:

4 cod fillets

2 tablespoons olive oil

1 lemon (sliced)

2 garlic cloves (minced)

1 tablespoon fresh parsley (chopped).

1 tablespoon fresh dill (chopped fresh dill-add to the potatoes and onions near the end of cooking).

When using the above ingredients, always remember to add a pinch of salt and pepper.

Instructions:

To start with, prepare your cooking space by heating the oven at 400°F (200°C).

Put the cod fillets into a baking tray and cover it with the parchment paper.

Pour a bit of olive oil over the top, then garnish with thin slices of lemon, minced garlic, fresh parsley, and dill.

Season with salt and pepper Season to taste with salt and pepper.

Cook them for about 15-20 minutes, until the fish turns opaque and can be easily flaked.

It is best served with steamed vegetables or even a simple fresh salad on the side.

Endometriosis Benefits: Cod is a low-profile fish that is loaded with lean protein and essential omega 3 fatty acids that have anti-inflammation properties. To bring out the nutritional value, the food has added fresh herbs accompanied by lemon which is rich in antioxidants.

Lentil and Vegetable Stew

Ingredients:

1 tablespoon olive oil

1 onion (chopped)

2 carrots (chopped)

2 celery stalks (chopped)

2 garlic cloves (minced)

1 cup dried lentils

1 can diced tomatoes

4 cups vegetable broth

1 teaspoon thyme

1 teaspoon rosemary

2 cups kale (chopped)

Then season with salt and/or black pepper if desired.

Instructions:

Coat the bottom of a large stock pot with olive oil, then turn the heat to medium.

Sauté the onion, carrots, and celery and put in the broth when they are semi-transparent.

Now pour garlic and sauté it for a minute.

Add lentils, tomatoes, vegetable stock and herbs: thyme, and rosemary into it.

Bring it to boil it, turn the heat low, and let it cook for 30-40 minutes, until lentil is soft.

It involves incorporating the kale into the mixture then stirring it until a wilted consistency is achieved.

Season with salt and pepper to your preference Let it cool slightly before.

Serve hot.

Endometriosis Benefits: It is notable that lentils are packed with protein and fiber-healthy nutrients that are beneficial for the human body. The vegetables included in the recipe offer nutritional value in form of vitamin, minerals, and antioxidants that are considered effective in tackling inflammation.

Grilled Chicken with Sweet Potato and Broccoli

Ingredients:

2 chicken breasts

1 tablespoon olive oil

2 sweet potatoes (boiled and cut into cubes)

2 cups broccoli florets

1 teaspoon paprika

1 teaspoon garlic powder

Season with salt and pepper to your desired liking.

Instructions:

Fire up the grill or a grill pan to medium-high heat.

Coat chicken breasts with paprika, garlic powder, salt and pepper.

Broil the chicken for about 6-8 minutes each side or until done.

In another pan, place olive oil and turn the heat to medium.

Add sweet potatoes and stir occasionally until they become soft and slightly caramelized, about 10-15 minutes.

Stir in the broccoli florets and continue to sauté for another 5-7 minutes until tender.

Grilled chicken with sweet potatoes and broccoli should be served.

Endometriosis Benefits: Chickens offer lean protein, while sweet potatoes are packed with beta-carotene and fiber. It contains sulforaphane that has anti-inflammatory effect.

Mediterranean Chickpea Salad

Ingredients:

1 can chickpeas (drained and rinsed)

1 cucumber (chopped)

1 cup cherry tomatoes, halved

¼ cup of red onion (chopped)

¼ cup Kalamata olives (sliced)

¼ cup feta cheese (optional)

2 tablespoons olive oil

1 tablespoon lemon juice

1 teaspoon dried oregano

Season with salt and pepper to taste

Instructions:

In a big bowl mix the chickpeas, cucumber, cherry tomatoes, red onion, olives, and feta cheese.

In a small bowl, combine the olive oil, lemon juice, oregano, salt and pepper.

Pour the dressing on the salad and mix gently.

Best served cold or at room temperature.

Endometriosis Benefits: This salad contains a lot of fiber and plant protein. Olive oil is rich in healthy fats while olives, cucumber, and tomatoes contain water and antioxidants respectively.

Snack Option

A simple yet delicious snack that combines something sweet with a natural nutrient-rich food is,

1. Fresh fruit and nut butter.

- Ingredients: Sliced apple or banana, 2 tablespoons almond or peanut butter Addition.

- Instructions: Eat apple and banana slices with nut butters for a fast and energizing meal.

2. Veggie sticks and Hummus Required Time: About an hour Equipment: A bowl, a spoon, a knife, a cutting board, and serving plates Preparation: Preparation involves preparing the hummus recipe and cutting the veggies into sticks.

- Ingredients: Carrots, cucumbers, bell peppers, 1 bowl of hummus.

- Instructions: It is very easy to prepare; accompany veggie sticks with Hummus for dipping.

3. Folded Paranthas and Sabudana Khichdi

- Ingredients: 2 Scoop low fat Greek yogurt, 1 tbsp mixed berries, 1 tbsp honey.

- Instructions: Enjoy yogurt with your favorite berries on the topping and add honey as a dressing to it.

4. Trail Mix

- Ingredients: 1/4 cup almonds, 1/4 cup walnuts, 1/4 cup dry cranberries and 1/4 cup dark chocolate chips.

- Instructions: Combine all ingredients in a bowl, making sure all the pieces of fruit are coated and then transfer the mixture to a resealable container.

Roasted Chickpeas

Ingredients:

We will need one can chickpeas, for which it is necessary to use drained and rinsed product.

1 tablespoon olive oil

1 teaspoon paprika

1/2 teaspoon garlic powder

1/2 teaspoon cumin

Salt to taste

Instructions:

First, prepare the vegetable by peeling the skin off and chopping it up into small pieces then set the oven at 400 degrees Fahrenheit (200 degrees Celsius).

Drying the chickpeas: Place the chickpeas in a paper towel and gently pat them in a bid to remove any moisture from the surface.

As for preparation, in a bowl, pour some olive oil and seasonings over the chickpeas.

Drain and place the chickpeas in a row on a baking tray, preferably in a single layer.

Pat the chickpeas and seasoning mix evenly onto a large baking sheet and roast for 20 to 30 minutes, tossing the pan once or twice with a fork halfway through to make sure the chickpeas are crispy.

Let cool before serving.

Endometriosis Benefits: Chickpeas are very nutritious since they are fairly rich in dietary fiber and plant protein. These spices bring Anti- inflammatory characteristics to the food you consume.

Nut and Seed Energy Balls

These protein-packed little balls incorporate some of the most potent sources of energy in the whole nut and seed kingdom.

Ingredients:

1 cup rolled oats

1/2 cup almond butter

Organic honey or organic maple syrup – 1/4 cup

1/4 cup flax seeds

1/4 cup chia seeds

Ingredients: 1/2 cup dark chocolate chips (I've used dairy-free chocolate chips to accommodate individuals with lactose intolerance).

1 teaspoon vanilla extract

Instructions:

In a large bowl, mix all the ingredients well.

Stir gently until powders are completely incorporated into the wet ingredients.

This mixture should then be rolled into small balls and then placed on a baking sheet.

Chill for at least 60 minutes prior to serving.

Endometriosis Benefits: This snack is protein-rich, contains healthy fats, and benefits from all the added fiber — a nutritious and tasty energy ball.

Avocado Hummus with Veggie Sticks

Ingredients:

1 ripe avocado

Possible triggers: Can of chickpeas (drained and rinsed)

2 tablespoons tahini

1 garlic clove (minced)

1 tablespoon olive oil

Juice of 1 lemon

As to the condiments, the salt and the pepper must be added according to the taste.

For example, an assortment of veggie sticks such as carrot, cucumber and bell pepper for use in dipping.

Instructions:

Throw all the ingredients to the food processor and pulse to blend – avocado, chickpeas, tahini, garlic, olive oil, and lemon juice, salt and pepper to taste.

Blend until smooth.

Serve with veggie sticks.

Endometriosis Benefits: This recipe of hummus is healthy because it contains avocado which is rich source of fatty acids and the chickpeas which provide fiber to the body in order to fighting inflammation of the blood vessels and stabilization of sugar in the body.

Apple Slices with almond butter

Ingredients:

1 apple (sliced)

2 tablespoons almond butter

Chopped almonds 1 tablespoon chia seeds (optional)

Instructions:

Peel the apple, remove the core and cut the fruit into thin slices.

On each slice of bread, spread a layer of almond butter.

Served with chia seeds if preferred.

Endometriosis Benefits: This means that Apples contain fiber and antioxidants while almond butter has proteins and healthy fats, therefore making it a perfect snack.

Greek Yogurt with Berries and Nuts

This is one of the most delicious recipes for making a healthy snack; and this is Greek Yogurt with Berries and Nuts.

Ingredients:

1 cup plain regular or low-fat Greek yogurt (can use dairy free yogurt if needed)

First, you need half a cup of mixed berries — blueberries, strawberries, raspberries.

Streusel: 2 tablespoons chopped nuts (almonds, walnuts, pecans)

1 teaspoon honey (optional)

Instructions:

Prepare a mixture of Greek yogurt, berries along with the nuts.

Pour a little honey on top if you wish.

Serve immediately.

Endometriosis Benefits: This sandwich is one of the healthiest meals you could eat because Greek yogurt is rich in protein and probiotics, and berries in antioxidants, while nuts contain healthful fats.

Edamame with Sea Salt

This delicacy simply known as Edamame with Sea Salt makes a perfect dish for a group of friends or even a family.

Ingredients:

To do this you will need 1 cup edamame preferably fresh but if you are lazy like me, frozen will also do.

1/2 teaspoon sea salt

Instructions:

If using frozen edamame, you should steam or boil it with the help of the instructions on the back of the pack.

Drain and sprinkle sea Salt over it.

Serve warm or chilled.

Endometriosis Benefits: Edamame is high in protein and fiber and that makes it a satiety-rich healthy snack for human consumption.

Chia Pudding

Ingredients:

1/4 cup chia seeds

Use 1 cup almond milk or any other dairy free milk of your choice.

1 teaspoon vanilla extract

1 tablespoon maple syrup

Additional fruit toppings for the dish (optional)

Instructions:

In a bowl, add chia seeds, almond milk, vanilla extract, and maple syrup into the mixing bowl.

Stir gently, allow it to settle for 5 minutes. Stir the mixture again to avoid formation of lumps that could impede the flow of electricity.

After that, cover and place in refrigerator for not less than 4 hours or better when left overnight.

Best served with fresh fruits on top of the dish.

Endometriosis Benefits: The chia seeds contain nutrients such as omega3 fatty acids, fiber, and antioxidants that assist in combating inflammation.

Kale Chips

Ingredients:

There should be one bunch of kale, but the leaves must be washed and dried before using.

1 tablespoon olive oil

1/2 teaspoon sea salt

Optional seasonings: 1 teaspoon onion powder 1/2 teaspoon garlic powder 1/2 teaspoon thyme

Instructions:

First, set the oven to required temperature of 350°F that is 175°C.

Before preparation, strip the kale of its stems, and then cut it into small pieces.

Kale: Place the washed kale in a large bowl and share it with olive oil, sea salt, and garlic powder.

Lay the kale flat on the baking sheet to roast in one flat layer to ensure even crisping.

There are many easy recipes for Arancini and here is one: Boil the rice in vegetable broth until tender and mix in Parmesan, butter, and chopped basil. When the shoes are cool enough to handle, remove the sole and empty the contents. They are a great snack for adults and children and have many other uses, such as: Oh well, to each their own – at least they were upfront about it. Serve the aranc

Let cool before serving.

Endometriosis Benefits: The children in the current study have increased their consumption of kale, which is a nutritionally valuable green vegetable with virus, mineral, and antioxidant content that is anti-inflammatory.

Healthy Living Tips for Endometriosis

Moreover, to optimisely manage and treat endometriosis, it requires creating a lifestyle that also includes dietary alterations and adopting different practices that can reduce the symptoms and enhance the quality of life. Here are some essential lifestyle tips to consider:Here are some essential lifestyle tips to consider:

The Management of Various Kinds of Stress

Stress and Endometriosis:

Stress causes a significant impact on hormones, thereby worsening the conditions associated with endometriosis including pain and other symptoms. There is always need to ensure that stress is well managed for one to have a better coping strategy with pain and enhanced quality of life.

Techniques:

1. Mindfulness Meditation:

- Description: There are diverse methods in practiced meditation, one of which is mindfulness, it is a process of paying attention to the present moment while avoiding any kind of judgement. This tendency can contribute to stress reduction and increase of reservists' emotional armor.

- How to Practice: You have to go to a comparatively quiet place, assume a comfortable position with your back straight and your feet flat on the floor, and then, close your eyes. Take some time now, if you will, to get a sense of your own breathing; simply pay attention to the in breath and the out breath. If you find yourself going to a different thought, secretly become aware that your focus has shifted and then take your mind back to your breathing.

2. Deep Breathing Exercises:

- Description: One common technique of achieving relaxation is deep or controlled breathing; this can help relax the muscles, slow down the heart rate and even ease indigestion.

- How to Practice: They should either sit or lie down comfortably on a surface of their own choosing. Take two pieces of paper, one put one in the chest and other put in the abdomen. Breathe in through the nose and feel the chest expand and the diaphragm drop, which allows the abdomen to expand. Breathe out with your mouth, but make sure you are taking only a small breath, and are not inhaling the smoke deeply into your lungs. Repeat for several minutes.

3. Yoga:

- Description: Yoga involves a series of physical exercises as well as certain positions, breathing techniques, and meditations to reduce stress and to increase the range of movements of the body.

- How to Practice: The simple measures that can be taken are the integration of daily or weekly yoga exercise regime. Avoid rigorous practices such as the Warrior Pose I or the Tree Pose and instead opt for lighter poses like the Child's Pose, the Cow Face Pose, and the Cat-Cow Pose.

4. Progressive Muscle Relaxation:

- Description: This technique involves contraction of muscles and later relaxation of the muscles in the system of the human body.

- How to Practice: First of all, tighten up the toes, then gradually move up the legs, the abdomen, back, arms, neck and head and then you have to relax every muscle for several seconds.

5. Journaling:

- Description: Most of the time, having emotions documented on paper can ease stress since a great deal of what goes on in our mind can be reassuring.

- How to Practice: For a few minutes each day, write about whatever feelings, thoughts, and experiences that you have collected throughout the day. The emphasis should be on the creativity because you are just required to write a message without worrying about spelling or punctuation.

Exercise and physical activities

Benefits of Exercise:

The physical exercise will help in easing the pain of endometriosis through increased circulation and removal of prostaglandins associated with inflammation and also through endorphins which act as body pain relievers.

Types of Exercise:

1. Low-Impact Aerobics:

- Examples: Exercise such as: walking; swimming; cycling; and many others.

- Benefits: Enhances he art health without great pressure placed on any part of the body.

2. Strength Training:

- Examples: push-ups, squats, leg press, dumb bells, resistance bands.

- Benefits: Strengthens muscles, which are essential in recommending support and maybe decrease pain accumulated.

3. Stretching and Flexibility Exercises:

- Examples: Pilates, gentle yoga, there are such interesting classes as pilates that help in the strengthening of the muscles of the abdomen and back.

- Benefits: It helps body adjust easily, relieves stiffness and aids in muscle movement.

4. Mind-Body Exercises:

- Examples: Tai chi, qigong Tai chi and qigong are another modern form of the ancient Chinese martial arts and is a set of gentle, flowing exercise that are practiced to improve the health.

- Benefits: Linking up both bodily activity and concentration is a handy way to fight off stress and be generally healthier.

Exercise Tips:

- Start Slowly: For anyone who is getting back into exercise after a period of inactivity or have never been active before it is advisable to begin the workout sessions with short periods and then gradually increase the length and difficulty of the workouts.

- Listen to Your Body: For example, do not try to force yourself to develop breakthrough ideas if your shoulders and neck are aching from hours at a computer. Take pleasures in activities you engage in, and change these as often as possible if necessary.

- Consistency: It is good to exercise on a sturdy basis, preferably with an average duration of 30 minutes most days in the week.

7. 3. resume: Why is sleep important?

Sleep and Endometriosis:

In conclusion, sleep is crucial for health and wellbeing, and the quality of sleep should therefore not be compromised. Lack of sleep might also deepen endometriosis by making it harder for the body to bear the pain and also decrease immune response.

Tips for Better Sleep:

1. Establish a Routine:

- Regular sleep schedule: get up at the same hour daily and also go to bed at the same time whether it is a working day or a weekend.

2. Create a Sleep-Friendly Environment:2. Create a Sleep-Friendly Environment:

- The bedroom should be cool with no light sources, and there should not be much noise either. Where possible, utilize blackout curtains and a white noise machine for effective disturbance control.

3. Limit Screen Time:

- Any use of smartphones or tablets or watching TV at least an hour before the time of going to bed should be discouraged because these have a tendency to emit blue light which presents a barrier to sleep.

4. Relax Before Bed:

- To avoid spending the night tossing and turning, establish a regular pre-sleep behavioral regimen that could include reading or taking a warm bath before going to bed.

5. Watch Your Diet:

- Reduce the size of their last meal of the day or have a heavy snack before going to bed, avoid caffeine-rich foods and drinks as well as alcohol before going to bed. As far as you are hungry at night, better to take a small meal than heave one.

7. Natural supplements can be drawn from plants that help body in various ways and they are natural so they do not pose a threat to the body Unlike chemicals supplements which are synthesized in laboratories they have some advantages, here are some of them.

Supplements for Endometriosis:

This article lists some of the supplements that may be useful in alleviating the symptoms of the disease and treating the underlying cause of inflammation, hormonal, and immunological dysfunction. Many supplements contain probiotics that help enhance digestion and improve gut or gastrointestinal health. As always, please consult your doctor before taking any new supplement.

Common Supplements:

1. Omega-3 Fatty Acids:

- Source: Wild salmon, rainbow trout, sardines, mackerel, herring, Atlantic herring, anchovies, chia seed, flaxseed oil, walnuts.

- Benefits: Some of the nutrients and compounds present in vegetables have been found to possess anti-inflammatory effects that might assist in managing inflammation and pain.

2. Turmeric (Curcumin):

- Source: Turmeric root, capsules, fine powder/or small particles below about 100 micrometers.

- Benefits: It has anti-inflammatory and antioxidant properties which when used may be of help in the management of endometriosis associated pain.

3. Vitamin D:

- Source: The two most common causes reported by the respondents are sun exposure and supplements.

- Benefits: Promotes immunity and has antioxidant effects that may decrease inflammation. Endometriosis is characterized by inflammation that occurs in areas of the body such as the pelvis and abdomen, and according to a study by Aprile et al 2016, patients who are inflicted with endometriosis suffer increased pain, especially if they have low vitamin D levels.

4. Magnesium:

- Source: That is why children can take supplements, eat green leaves and nuts.

- Benefits: It also assists in muscle relaxation and is effective in preventing or alleviating muscle cramps. Also, it can help improve sleep patterns as well as the general body and mental health.

5. Zinc:

- Source: Meats and seafood, nuts and seeds and supplements.

- Benefits: The rhizome aids the immune system by playing roles in tissue repair and inflammation.

6. Probiotics:

- Source: Yogurt, kefir, sauerkraut, kimchi – are classified as fermented foods and there are vitamin and mineral supplements.

- Benefits: That is widely used for improving the gut health, which is a key factor in the regulation of the immune system and inflammation.

Printed in Great Britain
by Amazon